THIS BOOK
belongs to:

Strain

Grower

Date

Acquired

$

| Indica | Hybrid | Sativa |

☐ Flower   ☐ Edible   ☐ Concentrate

Symptoms Relieved

Sweet
Fruity   Floral
Sour   Spicy
Earthy   Herbal
Woodsy

Notes

Effects	Strength
Peaceful	○ ○ ○ ○ ○
Sleepy	○ ○ ○ ○ ○
Pain Relief	○ ○ ○ ○ ○
Hungry	○ ○ ○ ○ ○
Uplifted	○ ○ ○ ○ ○
Creative	○ ○ ○ ○ ○

Ratings ☆ ☆ ☆ ☆ ☆

Strain

Grower

Date

Acquired

$

| Indica | Hybrid | Sativa |

☐ Flower ☐ Edible ☐ Concentrate

Symptoms Relieved

Sweet

Fruity

Floral

Sour

Spicy

Earthy

Herbal

Woodsy

Notes

Effects	Strength
Peaceful	○ ○ ○ ○ ○
Sleepy	○ ○ ○ ○ ○
Pain Relief	○ ○ ○ ○ ○
Hungry	○ ○ ○ ○ ○
Uplifted	○ ○ ○ ○ ○
Creative	○ ○ ○ ○ ○

Ratings ☆ ☆ ☆ ☆ ☆

Strain

Grower

Date

Acquired

$

| Indica | Hybrid | Sativa |

☐ Flower   ☐ Edible   ☐ Concentrate

Symptoms Relieved

Sweet
Fruity
Floral
Sour
Spicy
Earthy
Herbal
Woodsy

Notes

Effects	Strength
Peaceful	○ ○ ○ ○ ○
Sleepy	○ ○ ○ ○ ○
Pain Relief	○ ○ ○ ○ ○
Hungry	○ ○ ○ ○ ○
Uplifted	○ ○ ○ ○ ○
Creative	○ ○ ○ ○ ○

Ratings ☆ ☆ ☆ ☆ ☆

Strain

Grower

Date

Acquired

$

| Indica | Hybrid | Sativa |

☐ Flower　　☐ Edible　　☐ Concentrate

Symptoms Relieved

Sweet
Fruity　Floral
Sour　Spicy
Earthy　Herbal
Woodsy

Notes

Effects	Strength
Peaceful	○ ○ ○ ○ ○
Sleepy	○ ○ ○ ○ ○
Pain Relief	○ ○ ○ ○ ○
Hungry	○ ○ ○ ○ ○
Uplifted	○ ○ ○ ○ ○
Creative	○ ○ ○ ○ ○

Ratings ☆ ☆ ☆ ☆ ☆

Strain

Grower

Date

Acquired

$

| Indica | Hybrid | Sativa |

☐ Flower   ☐ Edible   ☐ Concentrate

Symptoms Relieved

Sweet

Fruity

Floral

Sour

Spicy

Earthy

Herbal

Woodsy

Notes

| Effects | Strength |

Peaceful ○ ○ ○ ○ ○

Sleepy ○ ○ ○ ○ ○

Pain Relief ○ ○ ○ ○ ○

Hungry ○ ○ ○ ○ ○

Uplifted ○ ○ ○ ○ ○

Creative ○ ○ ○ ○ ○

Ratings ☆ ☆ ☆ ☆ ☆

Strain

Grower

Date

Acquired

$

Indica	Hybrid	Sativa

☐ Flower   ☐ Edible   ☐ Concentrate

Symptoms Relieved

Sweet
Fruity
Floral
Sour
Spicy
Earthy
Herbal
Woodsy

Notes

Effects	**Strength**
Peaceful	○ ○ ○ ○ ○
Sleepy	○ ○ ○ ○ ○
Pain Relief	○ ○ ○ ○ ○
Hungry	○ ○ ○ ○ ○
Uplifted	○ ○ ○ ○ ○
Creative	○ ○ ○ ○ ○

Ratings ☆ ☆ ☆ ☆ ☆

Strain

Grower

Date

Acquired

$

| Indica | Hybrid | Sativa |

☐ Flower ☐ Edible ☐ Concentrate

Symptoms Relieved

Notes

Effects   **Strength**

Peaceful ○ ○ ○ ○ ○

Sleepy ○ ○ ○ ○ ○

Pain Relief ○ ○ ○ ○ ○

Hungry ○ ○ ○ ○ ○

Uplifted ○ ○ ○ ○ ○

Creative ○ ○ ○ ○ ○

Ratings ☆ ☆ ☆ ☆ ☆

Strain

Grower

Date

Acquired

$

| Indica | Hybrid | Sativa |

☐ Flower ☐ Edible ☐ Concentrate

Symptoms Relieved

Notes

Sweet

Fruity

Floral

Sour

Spicy

Earthy

Herbal

Woodsy

| **Effects** | **Strength** |

Peaceful ○ ○ ○ ○ ○

Sleepy ○ ○ ○ ○ ○

Pain Relief ○ ○ ○ ○ ○

Hungry ○ ○ ○ ○ ○

Uplifted ○ ○ ○ ○ ○

Creative ○ ○ ○ ○ ○

Ratings ☆ ☆ ☆ ☆ ☆

Strain

Grower

Date

Acquired

$

| Indica | Hybrid | Sativa |

☐ Flower ☐ Edible ☐ Concentrate

Symptoms Relieved

Sweet

Fruity

Floral

Sour

Spicy

Earthy

Herbal

Woodsy

Notes

| Effects | Strength |

Peaceful ○ ○ ○ ○ ○

Sleepy ○ ○ ○ ○ ○

Pain Relief ○ ○ ○ ○ ○

Hungry ○ ○ ○ ○ ○

Uplifted ○ ○ ○ ○ ○

Creative ○ ○ ○ ○ ○

Ratings ☆ ☆ ☆ ☆ ☆

Strain

Grower

Date

Acquired

$

| Indica | Hybrid | Sativa |

☐ Flower   ☐ Edible   ☐ Concentrate

Symptoms Relieved

Notes

Effects	Strength
Peaceful	○ ○ ○ ○ ○
Sleepy	○ ○ ○ ○ ○
Pain Relief	○ ○ ○ ○ ○
Hungry	○ ○ ○ ○ ○
Uplifted	○ ○ ○ ○ ○
Creative	○ ○ ○ ○ ○

Ratings ☆ ☆ ☆ ☆ ☆

Strain

Grower

Date

Acquired

$

| Indica | Hybrid | Sativa |

☐ Flower ☐ Edible ☐ Concentrate

Symptoms Relieved

Sweet

Fruity

Floral

Sour

Spicy

Earthy

Herbal

Woodsy

Notes

| **Effects** | **Strength** |

Peaceful ○ ○ ○ ○ ○

Sleepy ○ ○ ○ ○ ○

Pain Relief ○ ○ ○ ○ ○

Hungry ○ ○ ○ ○ ○

Uplifted ○ ○ ○ ○ ○

Creative ○ ○ ○ ○ ○

Ratings ☆ ☆ ☆ ☆ ☆

Strain

Grower

Date

Acquired

$

| Indica | Hybrid | Sativa |

☐ Flower ☐ Edible ☐ Concentrate

Symptoms Relieved

Sweet

Fruity

Floral

Sour

Spicy

Earthy

Herbal

Woodsy

Notes

Effects	Strength
Peaceful	○ ○ ○ ○ ○
Sleepy	○ ○ ○ ○ ○
Pain Relief	○ ○ ○ ○ ○
Hungry	○ ○ ○ ○ ○
Uplifted	○ ○ ○ ○ ○
Creative	○ ○ ○ ○ ○

Ratings ☆ ☆ ☆ ☆ ☆

Strain

Grower

Date

Acquired

$

| Indica | Hybrid | Sativa |

☐ Flower   ☐ Edible   ☐ Concentrate

Symptoms Relieved

Notes

Sweet

Fruity

Floral

Sour

Spicy

Earthy

Herbal

Woodsy

| **Effects** | **Strength** |

Peaceful ○ ○ ○ ○ ○

Sleepy ○ ○ ○ ○ ○

Pain Relief ○ ○ ○ ○ ○

Hungry ○ ○ ○ ○ ○

Uplifted ○ ○ ○ ○ ○

Creative ○ ○ ○ ○ ○

Ratings ☆ ☆ ☆ ☆ ☆

Strain

Grower

Date

Acquired

$

| Indica | Hybrid | Sativa |

☐ Flower ☐ Edible ☐ Concentrate

Symptoms Relieved

Sweet

Fruity

Floral

Sour

Spicy

Earthy

Herbal

Woodsy

Notes

Effects	Strength
Peaceful	○ ○ ○ ○ ○
Sleepy	○ ○ ○ ○ ○
Pain Relief	○ ○ ○ ○ ○
Hungry	○ ○ ○ ○ ○
Uplifted	○ ○ ○ ○ ○
Creative	○ ○ ○ ○ ○

Ratings ☆ ☆ ☆ ☆ ☆

Strain

Grower

Date

Acquired

$

| Indica | Hybrid | Sativa |

☐ Flower   ☐ Edible   ☐ Concentrate

Symptoms Relieved

Sweet

Fruity

Floral

Sour

Spicy

Earthy

Herbal

Woodsy

Notes

| **Effects** | **Strength** |

Peaceful

Sleepy

Pain Relief

Hungry

Uplifted

Creative

Ratings ☆ ☆ ☆ ☆ ☆

Strain

Grower

Date

Acquired

$

Indica	Hybrid	Sativa

☐ Flower ☐ Edible ☐ Concentrate

Symptoms Relieved

Sweet
Fruity
Floral
Sour
Spicy
Earthy
Herbal
Woodsy

Notes

Effects	Strength				
Peaceful	○	○	○	○	○
Sleepy	○	○	○	○	○
Pain Relief	○	○	○	○	○
Hungry	○	○	○	○	○
Uplifted	○	○	○	○	○
Creative	○	○	○	○	○

Ratings ☆ ☆ ☆ ☆ ☆

Strain

Grower

Date

Acquired

$

| Indica | Hybrid | Sativa |

☐ Flower ☐ Edible ☐ Concentrate

Symptoms Relieved

Sweet

Fruity

Floral

Sour

Spicy

Earthy

Herbal

Woodsy

Notes

Effects	Strength
Peaceful	○ ○ ○ ○ ○
Sleepy	○ ○ ○ ○ ○
Pain Relief	○ ○ ○ ○ ○
Hungry	○ ○ ○ ○ ○
Uplifted	○ ○ ○ ○ ○
Creative	○ ○ ○ ○ ○

Ratings ☆ ☆ ☆ ☆ ☆

Strain

Grower

Date

Acquired

$

| Indica | Hybrid | Sativa |

☐ Flower ☐ Edible ☐ Concentrate

Symptoms Relieved

Notes

Effects	Strength
Peaceful	○ ○ ○ ○ ○
Sleepy	○ ○ ○ ○ ○
Pain Relief	○ ○ ○ ○ ○
Hungry	○ ○ ○ ○ ○
Uplifted	○ ○ ○ ○ ○
Creative	○ ○ ○ ○ ○

Ratings ☆ ☆ ☆ ☆ ☆

Strain

Grower ___________________

Date ___________________

Acquired ___________________

$ ___________________

Indica	Hybrid	Sativa

☐ Flower   ☐ Edible   ☐ Concentrate

Symptoms Relieved

____
____
____
____

Notes

____
____
____
____
____
____
____

Effects	Strength				
Peaceful	○	○	○	○	○
Sleepy	○	○	○	○	○
Pain Relief	○	○	○	○	○
Hungry	○	○	○	○	○
Uplifted	○	○	○	○	○
Creative	○	○	○	○	○

Ratings ☆ ☆ ☆ ☆ ☆

Strain

Grower

Acquired

Date

$

| Indica | Hybrid | Sativa |

☐ Flower   ☐ Edible   ☐ Concentrate

Symptoms Relieved

Notes

Effects	**Strength**
Peaceful	○ ○ ○ ○ ○
Sleepy	○ ○ ○ ○ ○
Pain Relief	○ ○ ○ ○ ○
Hungry	○ ○ ○ ○ ○
Uplifted	○ ○ ○ ○ ○
Creative	○ ○ ○ ○ ○

Ratings ☆ ☆ ☆ ☆ ☆

Strain

Grower

Date

Acquired

$

| Indica | Hybrid | Sativa |

☐ Flower ☐ Edible ☐ Concentrate

Symptoms Relieved

Notes

Effects	Strength
Peaceful	○ ○ ○ ○ ○
Sleepy	○ ○ ○ ○ ○
Pain Relief	○ ○ ○ ○ ○
Hungry	○ ○ ○ ○ ○
Uplifted	○ ○ ○ ○ ○
Creative	○ ○ ○ ○ ○

Ratings ☆ ☆ ☆ ☆ ☆

Strain

Grower

Date

Acquired

$

| Indica | Hybrid | Sativa |

☐ Flower   ☐ Edible   ☐ Concentrate

Symptoms Relieved

Sweet
Fruity
Floral
Sour
Spicy
Earthy
Herbal
Woodsy

Notes

Effects	Strength
Peaceful	○ ○ ○ ○ ○
Sleepy	○ ○ ○ ○ ○
Pain Relief	○ ○ ○ ○ ○
Hungry	○ ○ ○ ○ ○
Uplifted	○ ○ ○ ○ ○
Creative	○ ○ ○ ○ ○

Ratings ☆ ☆ ☆ ☆ ☆

Strain

Grower ___________________________

Date ___________________________

Acquired ___________________________

$ ___________________________

Indica	Hybrid	Sativa

☐ Flower ☐ Edible ☐ Concentrate

Symptoms Relieved

____

____

____

____

____

Sweet

Fruity

Floral

Sour

Spicy

Earthy

Herbal

Woodsy

Notes

____

____

____

____

____

____

____

____

Effects	Strength				
Peaceful	○	○	○	○	○
Sleepy	○	○	○	○	○
Pain Relief	○	○	○	○	○
Hungry	○	○	○	○	○
Uplifted	○	○	○	○	○
Creative	○	○	○	○	○

Ratings ☆ ☆ ☆ ☆ ☆

Strain

Grower

Date

Acquired

$

| Indica | Hybrid | Sativa |

☐ Flower ☐ Edible ☐ Concentrate

Symptoms Relieved

Sweet
Fruity
Floral
Sour
Spicy
Earthy
Herbal
Woodsy

Notes

Effects	Strength
Peaceful	○ ○ ○ ○ ○
Sleepy	○ ○ ○ ○ ○
Pain Relief	○ ○ ○ ○ ○
Hungry	○ ○ ○ ○ ○
Uplifted	○ ○ ○ ○ ○
Creative	○ ○ ○ ○ ○

Ratings ☆ ☆ ☆ ☆ ☆

Strain

Grower

Date

Acquired

$

| Indica | Hybrid | Sativa |

☐ Flower ☐ Edible ☐ Concentrate

Symptoms Relieved

Notes

Sweet

Fruity

Floral

Sour

Spicy

Earthy

Herbal

Woodsy

Effects	Strength
Peaceful	◯ ◯ ◯ ◯ ◯
Sleepy	◯ ◯ ◯ ◯ ◯
Pain Relief	◯ ◯ ◯ ◯ ◯
Hungry	◯ ◯ ◯ ◯ ◯
Uplifted	◯ ◯ ◯ ◯ ◯
Creative	◯ ◯ ◯ ◯ ◯

Ratings ☆ ☆ ☆ ☆ ☆

Strain

Grower

Acquired

Date

$

Indica	Hybrid	Sativa

☐ Flower   ☐ Edible   ☐ Concentrate

Symptoms Relieved

Sweet
Fruity
Floral
Sour
Spicy
Earthy
Herbal
Woodsy

Notes

Effects	Strength				
Peaceful	○	○	○	○	○
Sleepy	○	○	○	○	○
Pain Relief	○	○	○	○	○
Hungry	○	○	○	○	○
Uplifted	○	○	○	○	○
Creative	○	○	○	○	○

Ratings ☆ ☆ ☆ ☆ ☆

Strain

Grower

Date

Acquired

$

| Indica | Hybrid | Sativa |

☐ Flower ☐ Edible ☐ Concentrate

Symptoms Relieved

Sweet

Fruity

Floral

Sour

Spicy

Earthy

Herbal

Woodsy

Notes

| **Effects** | **Strength** |

Peaceful ○ ○ ○ ○ ○

Sleepy ○ ○ ○ ○ ○

Pain Relief ○ ○ ○ ○ ○

Hungry ○ ○ ○ ○ ○

Uplifted ○ ○ ○ ○ ○

Creative ○ ○ ○ ○ ○

Ratings ☆ ☆ ☆ ☆ ☆

Strain

Grower

Date

Acquired

$

Indica	Hybrid	Sativa

☐ Flower   ☐ Edible   ☐ Concentrate

Symptoms Relieved

Sweet
Fruity
Floral
Sour
Spicy
Earthy
Herbal
Woodsy

Notes

Effects	Strength
Peaceful	○ ○ ○ ○ ○
Sleepy	○ ○ ○ ○ ○
Pain Relief	○ ○ ○ ○ ○
Hungry	○ ○ ○ ○ ○
Uplifted	○ ○ ○ ○ ○
Creative	○ ○ ○ ○ ○

Ratings ☆ ☆ ☆ ☆ ☆

Strain

Grower

Date

Acquired

$

| Indica | Hybrid | Sativa |

☐ Flower   ☐ Edible   ☐ Concentrate

Symptoms Relieved

Sweet

Fruity

Floral

Sour

Spicy

Earthy

Herbal

Woodsy

Notes

| **Effects** | **Strength** |

Peaceful ○ ○ ○ ○ ○

Sleepy ○ ○ ○ ○ ○

Pain Relief ○ ○ ○ ○ ○

Hungry ○ ○ ○ ○ ○

Uplifted ○ ○ ○ ○ ○

Creative ○ ○ ○ ○ ○

Ratings ☆ ☆ ☆ ☆ ☆

Strain

Grower

Date

Acquired

$

| Indica | Hybrid | Sativa |

☐ Flower   ☐ Edible   ☐ Concentrate

Symptoms Relieved

Notes

Sweet

Fruity

Floral

Sour

Spicy

Earthy

Herbal

Woodsy

Effects	**Strength**
Peaceful	◯ ◯ ◯ ◯ ◯
Sleepy	◯ ◯ ◯ ◯ ◯
Pain Relief	◯ ◯ ◯ ◯ ◯
Hungry	◯ ◯ ◯ ◯ ◯
Uplifted	◯ ◯ ◯ ◯ ◯
Creative	◯ ◯ ◯ ◯ ◯

Ratings ☆ ☆ ☆ ☆ ☆

Strain

Grower

Date

Acquired $

| Indica | Hybrid | Sativa |

☐ Flower ☐ Edible ☐ Concentrate

Symptoms Relieved

Sweet
Fruity
Floral
Sour
Spicy
Earthy
Herbal
Woodsy

Notes

Effects	Strength
Peaceful	○ ○ ○ ○ ○
Sleepy	○ ○ ○ ○ ○
Pain Relief	○ ○ ○ ○ ○
Hungry	○ ○ ○ ○ ○
Uplifted	○ ○ ○ ○ ○
Creative	○ ○ ○ ○ ○

Ratings ☆ ☆ ☆ ☆ ☆

Strain

____

Grower _______________________ Date _______________

Acquired _____________________ $ _______________

Indica	Hybrid	Sativa

☐ Flower   ☐ Edible   ☐ Concentrate

Symptoms Relieved

____
____
____
____

Notes

____
____
____
____
____
____
____

Effects	Strength				
Peaceful	○	○	○	○	○
Sleepy	○	○	○	○	○
Pain Relief	○	○	○	○	○
Hungry	○	○	○	○	○
Uplifted	○	○	○	○	○
Creative	○	○	○	○	○

Ratings ☆ ☆ ☆ ☆ ☆

Strain

Grower

Date

Acquired

$

| Indica | Hybrid | Sativa |

☐ Flower   ☐ Edible   ☐ Concentrate

Symptoms Relieved

Notes

Effects	Strength				
Peaceful	○	○	○	○	○
Sleepy	○	○	○	○	○
Pain Relief	○	○	○	○	○
Hungry	○	○	○	○	○
Uplifted	○	○	○	○	○
Creative	○	○	○	○	○

Ratings ☆ ☆ ☆ ☆ ☆

Strain

Grower

Date

Acquired

$

Indica	Hybrid	Sativa

☐ Flower ☐ Edible ☐ Concentrate

Symptoms Relieved

Notes

Sweet
Fruity
Floral
Sour
Spicy
Earthy
Herbal
Woodsy

Effects	Strength
Peaceful	○ ○ ○ ○ ○
Sleepy	○ ○ ○ ○ ○
Pain Relief	○ ○ ○ ○ ○
Hungry	○ ○ ○ ○ ○
Uplifted	○ ○ ○ ○ ○
Creative	○ ○ ○ ○ ○

Ratings ☆ ☆ ☆ ☆ ☆

Strain

Grower

Date

Acquired

$

| Indica | Hybrid | Sativa |

☐ Flower   ☐ Edible   ☐ Concentrate

Symptoms Relieved

Notes

Sweet
Fruity
Floral
Sour
Spicy
Earthy
Herbal
Woodsy

Effects	**Strength**
Peaceful	◯ ◯ ◯ ◯ ◯
Sleepy	◯ ◯ ◯ ◯ ◯
Pain Relief	◯ ◯ ◯ ◯ ◯
Hungry	◯ ◯ ◯ ◯ ◯
Uplifted	◯ ◯ ◯ ◯ ◯
Creative	◯ ◯ ◯ ◯ ◯

Ratings ☆ ☆ ☆ ☆ ☆

Strain

Grower

Date

Acquired

$

| Indica | Hybrid | Sativa |

☐ Flower   ☐ Edible   ☐ Concentrate

Symptoms Relieved

Notes

Effects	Strength
Peaceful	○ ○ ○ ○ ○
Sleepy	○ ○ ○ ○ ○
Pain Relief	○ ○ ○ ○ ○
Hungry	○ ○ ○ ○ ○
Uplifted	○ ○ ○ ○ ○
Creative	○ ○ ○ ○ ○

Ratings ☆ ☆ ☆ ☆ ☆

Strain

Grower

Date

Acquired

$

| Indica | Hybrid | Sativa |

☐ Flower ☐ Edible ☐ Concentrate

Symptoms Relieved

Notes

Effects	**Strength**
Peaceful	○ ○ ○ ○ ○
Sleepy	○ ○ ○ ○ ○
Pain Relief	○ ○ ○ ○ ○
Hungry	○ ○ ○ ○ ○
Uplifted	○ ○ ○ ○ ○
Creative	○ ○ ○ ○ ○

Ratings ☆ ☆ ☆ ☆ ☆

Strain

Grower

Date

Acquired

$

| Indica | Hybrid | Sativa |

☐ Flower   ☐ Edible   ☐ Concentrate

Symptoms Relieved

Notes

Sweet
Fruity
Floral
Sour
Spicy
Earthy
Herbal
Woodsy

Effects	**Strength**
Peaceful	○ ○ ○ ○ ○
Sleepy	○ ○ ○ ○ ○
Pain Relief	○ ○ ○ ○ ○
Hungry	○ ○ ○ ○ ○
Uplifted	○ ○ ○ ○ ○
Creative	○ ○ ○ ○ ○

Ratings ☆ ☆ ☆ ☆ ☆

Strain

Grower

Date

Acquired

$

| Indica | Hybrid | Sativa |

☐ Flower ☐ Edible ☐ Concentrate

Symptoms Relieved

Notes

Effects	Strength
Peaceful	○ ○ ○ ○ ○
Sleepy	○ ○ ○ ○ ○
Pain Relief	○ ○ ○ ○ ○
Hungry	○ ○ ○ ○ ○
Uplifted	○ ○ ○ ○ ○
Creative	○ ○ ○ ○ ○

Ratings ☆ ☆ ☆ ☆ ☆

Strain

Grower

Date

Acquired

$

Indica	Hybrid	Sativa

☐ Flower   ☐ Edible   ☐ Concentrate

Symptoms Relieved

Notes

Sweet

Fruity

Floral

Sour

Spicy

Earthy

Herbal

Woodsy

Effects	**Strength**
Peaceful	○ ○ ○ ○ ○
Sleepy	○ ○ ○ ○ ○
Pain Relief	○ ○ ○ ○ ○
Hungry	○ ○ ○ ○ ○
Uplifted	○ ○ ○ ○ ○
Creative	○ ○ ○ ○ ○

Ratings ☆ ☆ ☆ ☆ ☆

Strain

Grower

Date

Acquired

$

| Indica | Hybrid | Sativa |

☐ Flower   ☐ Edible   ☐ Concentrate

Symptoms Relieved

Sweet

Fruity

Floral

Sour

Spicy

Earthy

Herbal

Woodsy

Notes

Effects	Strength
Peaceful	○ ○ ○ ○ ○
Sleepy	○ ○ ○ ○ ○
Pain Relief	○ ○ ○ ○ ○
Hungry	○ ○ ○ ○ ○
Uplifted	○ ○ ○ ○ ○
Creative	○ ○ ○ ○ ○

Ratings ☆ ☆ ☆ ☆ ☆

Strain

Grower ______________________   Date ______________

Acquired ______________________ $ ______________

| Indica | Hybrid | Sativa |

☐ Flower   ☐ Edible   ☐ Concentrate

Symptoms Relieved

____

____

____

____

____

Sweet

Fruity   Floral

Sour   Spicy

Earthy   Herbal

Woodsy

Notes

____

____

____

____

____

____

____

Effects	**Strength**
Peaceful	○ ○ ○ ○ ○
Sleepy	○ ○ ○ ○ ○
Pain Relief	○ ○ ○ ○ ○
Hungry	○ ○ ○ ○ ○
Uplifted	○ ○ ○ ○ ○
Creative	○ ○ ○ ○ ○

Ratings ☆ ☆ ☆ ☆ ☆

Strain

Grower

Date

Acquired

$

| Indica | Hybrid | Sativa |

☐ Flower ☐ Edible ☐ Concentrate

Symptoms Relieved

Sweet
Fruity
Floral
Sour
Spicy
Earthy
Herbal
Woodsy

Notes

Effects	**Strength**
Peaceful	○ ○ ○ ○ ○
Sleepy	○ ○ ○ ○ ○
Pain Relief	○ ○ ○ ○ ○
Hungry	○ ○ ○ ○ ○
Uplifted	○ ○ ○ ○ ○
Creative	○ ○ ○ ○ ○

Ratings ☆ ☆ ☆ ☆ ☆

Strain

Grower

Date

Acquired

$

| Indica | Hybrid | Sativa |

☐ Flower ☐ Edible ☐ Concentrate

Symptoms Relieved

Notes

Effects	Strength
Peaceful	○ ○ ○ ○ ○
Sleepy	○ ○ ○ ○ ○
Pain Relief	○ ○ ○ ○ ○
Hungry	○ ○ ○ ○ ○
Uplifted	○ ○ ○ ○ ○
Creative	○ ○ ○ ○ ○

Ratings ☆ ☆ ☆ ☆ ☆

Strain

Grower

Date

Acquired

$

| Indica | Hybrid | Sativa |

☐ Flower   ☐ Edible   ☐ Concentrate

Symptoms Relieved

Notes

Effects   **Strength**

Peaceful ○ ○ ○ ○ ○

Sleepy ○ ○ ○ ○ ○

Pain Relief ○ ○ ○ ○ ○

Hungry ○ ○ ○ ○ ○

Uplifted ○ ○ ○ ○ ○

Creative ○ ○ ○ ○ ○

Ratings ☆ ☆ ☆ ☆ ☆

Strain

Grower

Date

Acquired

$

| Indica | Hybrid | Sativa |

☐ Flower ☐ Edible ☐ Concentrate

Symptoms Relieved

Sweet
Fruity
Floral
Sour
Spicy
Earthy
Herbal
Woodsy

Notes

Effects	Strength
Peaceful	○ ○ ○ ○ ○
Sleepy	○ ○ ○ ○ ○
Pain Relief	○ ○ ○ ○ ○
Hungry	○ ○ ○ ○ ○
Uplifted	○ ○ ○ ○ ○
Creative	○ ○ ○ ○ ○

Ratings ☆ ☆ ☆ ☆ ☆

Strain

Grower

Date

Acquired

$

Indica	Hybrid	Sativa

☐ Flower ☐ Edible ☐ Concentrate

Symptoms Relieved

Sweet
Fruity
Floral
Sour
Spicy
Earthy
Herbal
Woodsy

Notes

Effects	Strength
Peaceful	○ ○ ○ ○ ○
Sleepy	○ ○ ○ ○ ○
Pain Relief	○ ○ ○ ○ ○
Hungry	○ ○ ○ ○ ○
Uplifted	○ ○ ○ ○ ○
Creative	○ ○ ○ ○ ○

Ratings ☆ ☆ ☆ ☆ ☆

Strain

Grower

Date

Acquired

$

| Indica | Hybrid | Sativa |

☐ Flower ☐ Edible ☐ Concentrate

Symptoms Relieved

Notes

| Effects | Strength |

Peaceful ○ ○ ○ ○ ○

Sleepy ○ ○ ○ ○ ○

Pain Relief ○ ○ ○ ○ ○

Hungry ○ ○ ○ ○ ○

Uplifted ○ ○ ○ ○ ○

Creative ○ ○ ○ ○ ○

Ratings ☆ ☆ ☆ ☆ ☆

Strain

Grower

Date

Acquired

$

| Indica | Hybrid | Sativa |

☐ Flower   ☐ Edible   ☐ Concentrate

Symptoms Relieved

Sweet
Fruity
Floral
Sour
Spicy
Earthy
Herbal
Woodsy

Notes

Effects	Strength
Peaceful	○ ○ ○ ○ ○
Sleepy	○ ○ ○ ○ ○
Pain Relief	○ ○ ○ ○ ○
Hungry	○ ○ ○ ○ ○
Uplifted	○ ○ ○ ○ ○
Creative	○ ○ ○ ○ ○

Ratings ☆ ☆ ☆ ☆ ☆

Strain

Grower

Date

Acquired

$

| Indica | Hybrid | Sativa |

☐ Flower   ☐ Edible   ☐ Concentrate

Symptoms Relieved

Notes

Sweet

Fruity

Floral

Sour

Spicy

Earthy

Herbal

Woodsy

| **Effects** | **Strength** |

Peaceful ○ ○ ○ ○ ○

Sleepy ○ ○ ○ ○ ○

Pain Relief ○ ○ ○ ○ ○

Hungry ○ ○ ○ ○ ○

Uplifted ○ ○ ○ ○ ○

Creative ○ ○ ○ ○ ○

Ratings ☆ ☆ ☆ ☆ ☆

Strain

Grower

Date

Acquired

$

| Indica | Hybrid | Sativa |

☐ Flower   ☐ Edible   ☐ Concentrate

Symptoms Relieved

Sweet
Fruity · Floral
Sour · Spicy
Earthy · Herbal
Woodsy

Notes

Effects	Strength
Peaceful	○ ○ ○ ○ ○
Sleepy	○ ○ ○ ○ ○
Pain Relief	○ ○ ○ ○ ○
Hungry	○ ○ ○ ○ ○
Uplifted	○ ○ ○ ○ ○
Creative	○ ○ ○ ○ ○

Ratings ☆ ☆ ☆ ☆ ☆

Strain

Grower

Acquired

Date

$

Indica	Hybrid	Sativa

☐ Flower   ☐ Edible   ☐ Concentrate

Symptoms Relieved

Sweet

Fruity

Floral

Sour

Spicy

Earthy

Herbal

Woodsy

Notes

Effects	Strength				
Peaceful	○	○	○	○	○
Sleepy	○	○	○	○	○
Pain Relief	○	○	○	○	○
Hungry	○	○	○	○	○
Uplifted	○	○	○	○	○
Creative	○	○	○	○	○

Ratings ☆ ☆ ☆ ☆ ☆

Strain

Grower ____________________ Date ____________

Acquired ____________________ $ ____________

Indica	Hybrid	Sativa

☐ Flower   ☐ Edible   ☐ Concentrate

Symptoms Relieved

____

____

____

____

____

Notes

____

____

____

____

____

____

____

____

Effects	Strength				
Peaceful	○	○	○	○	○
Sleepy	○	○	○	○	○
Pain Relief	○	○	○	○	○
Hungry	○	○	○	○	○
Uplifted	○	○	○	○	○
Creative	○	○	○	○	○

Ratings ☆ ☆ ☆ ☆ ☆

Strain

Grower ______________________   Date ______________

Acquired ______________________ $ ______________

Indica	Hybrid	Sativa

☐ Flower   ☐ Edible   ☐ Concentrate

Symptoms Relieved

____

____

____

____

____

Sweet

Fruity

Floral

Sour

Spicy

Earthy

Herbal

Woodsy

Notes

____

____

____

____

____

____

____

Effects	Strength				
Peaceful	◯	◯	◯	◯	◯
Sleepy	◯	◯	◯	◯	◯
Pain Relief	◯	◯	◯	◯	◯
Hungry	◯	◯	◯	◯	◯
Uplifted	◯	◯	◯	◯	◯
Creative	◯	◯	◯	◯	◯

Ratings ☆ ☆ ☆ ☆ ☆

Strain

Grower _______________________   Date _______________________

Acquired _______________________ $ _______________________

Indica	Hybrid	Sativa

☐ Flower   ☐ Edible   ☐ Concentrate

Symptoms Relieved

Notes

Effects	Strength				
Peaceful	○	○	○	○	○
Sleepy	○	○	○	○	○
Pain Relief	○	○	○	○	○
Hungry	○	○	○	○	○
Uplifted	○	○	○	○	○
Creative	○	○	○	○	○

Ratings ☆ ☆ ☆ ☆ ☆

Strain

Grower ___________________________ Date ___________________

Acquired _________________________ $ ______________________

Indica	Hybrid	Sativa

☐ Flower   ☐ Edible   ☐ Concentrate

Symptoms Relieved

____

____

____

____

Sweet
Fruity
Floral
Sour
Spicy
Earthy
Herbal
Woodsy

Notes

____

____

____

____

____

____

____

Effects	Strength				
Peaceful	○	○	○	○	○
Sleepy	○	○	○	○	○
Pain Relief	○	○	○	○	○
Hungry	○	○	○	○	○
Uplifted	○	○	○	○	○
Creative	○	○	○	○	○

Ratings ☆ ☆ ☆ ☆ ☆

Strain

Grower

Date

Acquired

$

| Indica | Hybrid | Sativa |

☐ Flower   ☐ Edible   ☐ Concentrate

Symptoms Relieved

Sweet
Fruity
Floral
Sour
Spicy
Earthy
Herbal
Woodsy

Notes

Effects	**Strength**
Peaceful	○ ○ ○ ○ ○
Sleepy	○ ○ ○ ○ ○
Pain Relief	○ ○ ○ ○ ○
Hungry	○ ○ ○ ○ ○
Uplifted	○ ○ ○ ○ ○
Creative	○ ○ ○ ○ ○

Ratings ☆ ☆ ☆ ☆ ☆

Strain

Grower

Date

Acquired

$

| Indica | Hybrid | Sativa |

☐ Flower ☐ Edible ☐ Concentrate

Symptoms Relieved

Sweet
Fruity
Floral
Sour
Spicy
Earthy
Herbal
Woodsy

Notes

Effects	Strength
Peaceful	○ ○ ○ ○ ○
Sleepy	○ ○ ○ ○ ○
Pain Relief	○ ○ ○ ○ ○
Hungry	○ ○ ○ ○ ○
Uplifted	○ ○ ○ ○ ○
Creative	○ ○ ○ ○ ○

Ratings ☆ ☆ ☆ ☆ ☆

Strain

Grower

Date

Acquired

$

| Indica | Hybrid | Sativa |

☐ Flower   ☐ Edible   ☐ Concentrate

Symptoms Relieved

Notes

Effects	**Strength**
Peaceful	○ ○ ○ ○ ○
Sleepy	○ ○ ○ ○ ○
Pain Relief	○ ○ ○ ○ ○
Hungry	○ ○ ○ ○ ○
Uplifted	○ ○ ○ ○ ○
Creative	○ ○ ○ ○ ○

Ratings ☆ ☆ ☆ ☆ ☆

Strain

Grower

Date

Acquired $

| Indica | Hybrid | Sativa |

☐ Flower   ☐ Edible   ☐ Concentrate

Symptoms Relieved

Notes

Sweet
Fruity   Floral
Sour   Spicy
Earthy   Herbal
Woodsy

Effects	**Strength**				
Peaceful	○	○	○	○	○
Sleepy	○	○	○	○	○
Pain Relief	○	○	○	○	○
Hungry	○	○	○	○	○
Uplifted	○	○	○	○	○
Creative	○	○	○	○	○

Ratings ☆ ☆ ☆ ☆ ☆

Strain

Grower

Date

Acquired

$

Indica | Hybrid | Sativa

☐ Flower   ☐ Edible   ☐ Concentrate

Symptoms Relieved

Sweet
Fruity
Floral
Sour
Spicy
Earthy
Herbal
Woodsy

Notes

Effects	Strength
Peaceful	○ ○ ○ ○ ○
Sleepy	○ ○ ○ ○ ○
Pain Relief	○ ○ ○ ○ ○
Hungry	○ ○ ○ ○ ○
Uplifted	○ ○ ○ ○ ○
Creative	○ ○ ○ ○ ○

Ratings ☆ ☆ ☆ ☆ ☆

Strain

Grower

Date

Acquired

$

| Indica | Hybrid | Sativa |

☐ Flower ☐ Edible ☐ Concentrate

Symptoms Relieved

Sweet
Fruity
Floral
Sour
Spicy
Earthy
Herbal
Woodsy

Notes

Effects	Strength
Peaceful	○ ○ ○ ○ ○
Sleepy	○ ○ ○ ○ ○
Pain Relief	○ ○ ○ ○ ○
Hungry	○ ○ ○ ○ ○
Uplifted	○ ○ ○ ○ ○
Creative	○ ○ ○ ○ ○

Ratings ☆ ☆ ☆ ☆ ☆

Strain

Grower

Date

Acquired

$

| Indica | Hybrid | Sativa |

☐ Flower ☐ Edible ☐ Concentrate

Symptoms Relieved

Sweet
Fruity
Floral
Sour
Spicy
Earthy
Herbal
Woodsy

Notes

Effects	Strength
Peaceful	○ ○ ○ ○ ○
Sleepy	○ ○ ○ ○ ○
Pain Relief	○ ○ ○ ○ ○
Hungry	○ ○ ○ ○ ○
Uplifted	○ ○ ○ ○ ○
Creative	○ ○ ○ ○ ○

Ratings ☆ ☆ ☆ ☆ ☆

Strain

Grower

Acquired

Date

$

| Indica | Hybrid | Sativa |

☐ Flower ☐ Edible ☐ Concentrate

Symptoms Relieved

Sweet
Fruity
Floral
Sour
Spicy
Earthy
Herbal
Woodsy

Notes

Effects	**Strength**
Peaceful	○ ○ ○ ○ ○
Sleepy	○ ○ ○ ○ ○
Pain Relief	○ ○ ○ ○ ○
Hungry	○ ○ ○ ○ ○
Uplifted	○ ○ ○ ○ ○
Creative	○ ○ ○ ○ ○

Ratings ☆ ☆ ☆ ☆ ☆

Strain

Grower

Date

Acquired

$

| Indica | Hybrid | Sativa |

☐ Flower ☐ Edible ☐ Concentrate

Symptoms Relieved

Notes

Sweet
Fruity
Floral
Sour
Spicy
Earthy
Herbal
Woodsy

Effects	Strength
Peaceful	○ ○ ○ ○ ○
Sleepy	○ ○ ○ ○ ○
Pain Relief	○ ○ ○ ○ ○
Hungry	○ ○ ○ ○ ○
Uplifted	○ ○ ○ ○ ○
Creative	○ ○ ○ ○ ○

Ratings ☆ ☆ ☆ ☆ ☆

Strain

Grower

Date

Acquired

$

| Indica | Hybrid | Sativa |

☐ Flower ☐ Edible ☐ Concentrate

Symptoms Relieved

Notes

Effects	Strength
Peaceful	○ ○ ○ ○ ○
Sleepy	○ ○ ○ ○ ○
Pain Relief	○ ○ ○ ○ ○
Hungry	○ ○ ○ ○ ○
Uplifted	○ ○ ○ ○ ○
Creative	○ ○ ○ ○ ○

Ratings ☆ ☆ ☆ ☆ ☆

Strain

Grower __________________________   Date __________

Acquired __________________________ $ __________

| Indica | Hybrid | Sativa |

☐ Flower   ☐ Edible   ☐ Concentrate

Symptoms Relieved

Notes

Sweet · Fruity · Floral · Sour · Spicy · Earthy · Herbal · Woodsy

Effects	Strength
Peaceful	○ ○ ○ ○ ○
Sleepy	○ ○ ○ ○ ○
Pain Relief	○ ○ ○ ○ ○
Hungry	○ ○ ○ ○ ○
Uplifted	○ ○ ○ ○ ○
Creative	○ ○ ○ ○ ○

Ratings ☆ ☆ ☆ ☆ ☆

Strain

Grower

Date

Acquired

$

| Indica | Hybrid | Sativa |

☐ Flower ☐ Edible ☐ Concentrate

Symptoms Relieved

Notes

Effects	Strength
Peaceful	○ ○ ○ ○ ○
Sleepy	○ ○ ○ ○ ○
Pain Relief	○ ○ ○ ○ ○
Hungry	○ ○ ○ ○ ○
Uplifted	○ ○ ○ ○ ○
Creative	○ ○ ○ ○ ○

Ratings ☆ ☆ ☆ ☆ ☆

Strain

Grower ______________________

Date ______________________

Acquired ______________________

$ ______________________

| Indica | Hybrid | Sativa |

☐ Flower ☐ Edible ☐ Concentrate

Symptoms Relieved

Sweet

Fruity

Floral

Sour

Spicy

Earthy

Herbal

Woodsy

Notes

Effects	Strength
Peaceful	○ ○ ○ ○ ○
Sleepy	○ ○ ○ ○ ○
Pain Relief	○ ○ ○ ○ ○
Hungry	○ ○ ○ ○ ○
Uplifted	○ ○ ○ ○ ○
Creative	○ ○ ○ ○ ○

Ratings ☆ ☆ ☆ ☆ ☆

Strain

Grower

Date

Acquired

$

| Indica | Hybrid | Sativa |

☐ Flower   ☐ Edible   ☐ Concentrate

Symptoms Relieved

Sweet

Fruity

Floral

Sour

Spicy

Earthy

Herbal

Woodsy

Notes

Effects	Strength
Peaceful	○ ○ ○ ○ ○
Sleepy	○ ○ ○ ○ ○
Pain Relief	○ ○ ○ ○ ○
Hungry	○ ○ ○ ○ ○
Uplifted	○ ○ ○ ○ ○
Creative	○ ○ ○ ○ ○

Ratings ☆ ☆ ☆ ☆ ☆

Strain

Grower ___________________________ Date ___________________

Acquired _________________________ $ ______________________

| Indica | Hybrid | Sativa |

☐ Flower   ☐ Edible   ☐ Concentrate

Symptoms Relieved

____

____

____

____

Notes

____

____

____

____

____

____

____

____

Effects	**Strength**				
Peaceful	○	○	○	○	○
Sleepy	○	○	○	○	○
Pain Relief	○	○	○	○	○
Hungry	○	○	○	○	○
Uplifted	○	○	○	○	○
Creative	○	○	○	○	○

Ratings ☆ ☆ ☆ ☆ ☆

Strain

Grower

Date

Acquired

$

| Indica | Hybrid | Sativa |

☐ Flower ☐ Edible ☐ Concentrate

Symptoms Relieved

Notes

Sweet

Fruity

Floral

Sour

Spicy

Earthy

Herbal

Woodsy

Effects	**Strength**
Peaceful	○ ○ ○ ○ ○
Sleepy	○ ○ ○ ○ ○
Pain Relief	○ ○ ○ ○ ○
Hungry	○ ○ ○ ○ ○
Uplifted	○ ○ ○ ○ ○
Creative	○ ○ ○ ○ ○

Ratings ☆ ☆ ☆ ☆ ☆

Strain

Grower

Date

Acquired

$

| Indica | Hybrid | Sativa |

☐ Flower   ☐ Edible   ☐ Concentrate

Symptoms Relieved

Notes

Effects	Strength
Peaceful	○ ○ ○ ○ ○
Sleepy	○ ○ ○ ○ ○
Pain Relief	○ ○ ○ ○ ○
Hungry	○ ○ ○ ○ ○
Uplifted	○ ○ ○ ○ ○
Creative	○ ○ ○ ○ ○

Ratings ☆ ☆ ☆ ☆ ☆

Strain

Grower

Date

Acquired

$

Indica	Hybrid	Sativa

☐ Flower   ☐ Edible   ☐ Concentrate

Symptoms Relieved

Notes

Effects	Strength				
Peaceful	○	○	○	○	○
Sleepy	○	○	○	○	○
Pain Relief	○	○	○	○	○
Hungry	○	○	○	○	○
Uplifted	○	○	○	○	○
Creative	○	○	○	○	○

Ratings ☆ ☆ ☆ ☆ ☆

Strain

Grower

Date

Acquired

$

| Indica | Hybrid | Sativa |

☐ Flower   ☐ Edible   ☐ Concentrate

Symptoms Relieved

Notes

Sweet
Fruity
Floral
Sour
Spicy
Earthy
Herbal
Woodsy

Effects	Strength
Peaceful	○ ○ ○ ○ ○
Sleepy	○ ○ ○ ○ ○
Pain Relief	○ ○ ○ ○ ○
Hungry	○ ○ ○ ○ ○
Uplifted	○ ○ ○ ○ ○
Creative	○ ○ ○ ○ ○

Ratings ☆ ☆ ☆ ☆ ☆

Strain

Grower

Date

Acquired

$

| Indica | Hybrid | Sativa |

☐ Flower   ☐ Edible   ☐ Concentrate

Symptoms Relieved

Notes

Sweet

Fruity   Floral

Sour   Spicy

Earthy   Herbal

Woodsy

Effects	Strength
Peaceful	○ ○ ○ ○ ○
Sleepy	○ ○ ○ ○ ○
Pain Relief	○ ○ ○ ○ ○
Hungry	○ ○ ○ ○ ○
Uplifted	○ ○ ○ ○ ○
Creative	○ ○ ○ ○ ○

Ratings ☆ ☆ ☆ ☆ ☆